Table of Contents

EASIEST WAY TO STOP SMOKING

Please feel free to continue to smoke until you finish this book.

Welcome to "Easiest Way To Stop Smoking".

You now hold in your hands a book that **without a shadow of a doubt** will change your life! Indeed, if you use this book exactly as instructed, you **cannot fail** to achieve your goal of becoming a non smoker! How can I make such a powerful claim? Do yourself a favor and find out by reading this book from cover to cover!

Now without further ado, let's get straight down to business. There is only one reason you are still a smoker and it is this:

You are constantly in the grip of a psychological process called denial.

INTRODUCTION

Until you gain an awareness of this denial process you will find it difficult, if not impossible, to stop smoking. This book will teach you how to recognise and deal with your denial and will equip you with all the knowledge and skills that you will need to become a non smoker. On completion of the book and its tasks, you will feel much more in control and will be in a position of such power that you will actively welcome the stop smoking challenge.

1- YOU AS A SMOKER

Permanently stale breath, morning phlegm cough, nicotine stained teeth, shorter life expectancy, stained fingers, constant financial drain, various health problems, poor role model for your kids, dirty ashtrays, bland tasting food, smelly clothes and more and more frequently in today's health conscious climate, a lack of social acceptance.

2- YOU AS A NON SMOKER

Fresher breath, cleaner lungs, whiter teeth, likely to live longer, no stains on your fingers, more money, better all round health, good role model for your kids, tastier food, fresher home, fresher clothes and a greater level of social acceptability.

These two very different images serve to highlight the fact that if you are prepared to tolerate all these negative aspects of smoking, ie., the health risks, the cost, the stale odors etc., then you really must be getting something very powerful indeed in return. Furthermore, if you consider that you continually pay for your need to smoke, not just with money, but also with part of your life expectancy, and with some of your potential for good health, then it is easy to see that you are not just smoking for pleasure, or because you like the taste, or because it gives you something to do with your hands. The truth of the matter is this - you are prepared to pay such a huge price to continue smoking because you are **addicted** to the chemical nicotine.

Even if you don't think that you are addicted to nicotine, please bear with me until you get to the section on addiction. You might find that it is your **denial** that doesn't allow you to see that you are addicted. Denial is an integral part of the addiction condition and without understanding how your own denial process works; you will find it very difficult to overcome your desire to smoke.

This book is centrally focused around this process, and will teach you everything you need to know about denial, in order that you can be ready to deal with it when it attacks.

Who exactly is this book for?

This book is designed for everyone who seriously wants to stop smoking.

It doesn't matter if you are a five a day teenager, or a one hundred a day pensioner, male or female, or if this is your first or fiftieth attempt at stopping - if you really want to stop smoking then this is the book for you. Here's why:

The addiction perspective:

Because this book tackles smoking from an addiction perspective, it recognizes that you will repeatedly face both psychological and physical withdrawal difficulties.

You will learn as you progress through each chapter how to deal effectively with such difficulties and will find that stopping smoking will not be as difficult as you might previously have thought or experienced.

The information that follows will allow you to stop smoking with only a small and completely manageable level of discomfort, and will focus in the main on the absolute core of your addiction - your denial mechanism.

Later on you will be looking at this denial process in some depth, but in the mean time here is some basic information on how your denial works:

There is a little piece of your unconscious mind (the bit of your mind that thinks without you being aware of it) that will constantly try to trick you into smoking. It will do this by either,

(A) Making you feel that nicotine withdrawal is unbearable and that stopping smoking is not worth the discomfort and effort. Or by,

(B) Creating what seems to your conscious mind (the bit that you think with and *are* aware of) like really good reasons for starting smoking again.

It achieves this by passing these invented 'reasons' to your conscious mind in the form of a thought or an idea. For example, having made the decision to stop smoking, you might find yourself a few hours later thinking "Actually, now that I come to think of it, this isn't really a good time to stop - I think I'll stop next week instead when I'm not under so much pressure".

With the help of this book you will soon learn that these 'reasons' created by your unconscious mind are _always_ nonsense. On closer examination they will be   exposed   as   a   mechanism   that   allows   you   to   resume smoking, by giving you a guilt reducing excuse that you can use to justify your change of heart.

More importantly, these reasons give you the excuse you need to smoke, and smoking will, of course, relieve your unpleasant feelings of withdrawal. This is exactly what denial is all about - it is your unconscious mind finding any excuse at all, no matter how ridiculous, that will allow you to justify smoking, and thereby relieve your feelings of discomfort.

Your denial will be able to create excuse after excuse, and will convince you that these excuses are all completely plausible. Reasons, perhaps, like:

"If it hadn't been for that boss of mine embarrassing me in front of my work mates....", or, "If only I hadn't been caught speeding....", or, "if my boyfriend hadn't split up with me....", or, "It's my birthday next month, perhaps I'll wait until then to stop....", or any one of a thousand other rationalizations or justifications, every single one of which, if believed, will ensure your failure. The real reason you continue to smoke (not the one created by your unconscious) is simply this:

YOU DO NOT LIKE THE FEELINGS OF WITHDRAWAL

This book can, and will, create in you an awareness which will allow you to override this destructive unconscious 'voice' and will give you the tools you need to look honestly at the pain of withdrawal. It will help you to see that most of your discomfort is in fact an illusion, created deliberately by your unconscious.

Once you have learned how to tackle the discomfort of withdrawal and discovered how to recognize and defeat that ever present destructive unconscious 'voice', you will then move on to tackling associated difficulties such as unwanted weight gain. You will then learn how to set up effective support structures to help ensure your long term success.

In the final section, you will find an easy to follow 'battle plan', summarising all of the support strategies discussed in the book.

In some sections of the book there will be exercises to help you to understand the addiction process and how you are affected by it, and also how to deal simply and effectively with each potential relapse situation as it arises.

What this book isn't:

This book is not going to try to scare you into stopping smoking by telling you that if you don't stop you will **die** younger, or that you are much more likely to get cancer or some other smoking related disease. Let's face it - you already know all that scary health stuff and you are still a smoker! Scare tactics simply don't work!

Another thing this book won't be asking you to do is to reduce your smoking over a period of time with a view to eventually stopping altogether. This tactic is common, but usually ineffective. Reducing nicotine intake slowly still keeps your body supplied with at least some nicotine, right up to the point where you stop smoking altogether and your withdrawal symptoms begin.

This process is ineffective when you consider that at the end of your cutting down period you are still going to be plunged headlong into the difficulty of dealing with withdrawal. Why bother? You can start dealing with being a non smoker as soon as you finish this book, without having to torture yourself for weeks beforehand!

Your newly acquired skills and knowledge really will give you the edge that you need to stop smoking without too much difficulty and will allow you to start your new life as a non smoker immediately. Although the cutting down method may work for a few people, experience has shown that the most effective method of stopping smoking is to simply stop, then deal with any issues that may arise.

The method of stopping smoking discussed in this book is undoubtedly effective. It is also realistic. It doesn't promise you a totally pain free ride. It does though; teach you how to effectively manage the discomfort of withdrawal. You have, I'm sure, heard talk of the 'easy' way to stop smoking - wishful thinking I'm afraid! If stopping smoking was easy then surely just about everyone who smokes would have already stopped!

The method discussed in this book works, because it recognizes the fact that you are addicted to nicotine and therefore your solution must lie in Dealing with the physical and psychological problems that nicotine addiction presents.

This addiction / denial centered approach really does work and, it is absolutely guaranteed to work for you, providing that you take all the lessons to heart and follow all instructions to the letter. If you are prepared to do this then you will gain something that you really want - you will become a non smoker! Of course, like just about everything in life that is worth having, it does not come for free - you are going to have to pay a price!

That price is as follows:

1- You must agree to participate fully in all the exercises.

2- You must agree to pay the price of feeling at least *some* discomfort, *some* of the time.

3- You must agree to *use* the knowledge and skills in this book to overcome any withdrawal discomfort that you might feel.

4- You must agree to follow all instructions. *Even if you can't always see the point!*

Now, if you can agree to all of these simple terms then, as I mentioned earlier, I am prepared to offer you this guarantee:

I <u>absolutely</u> guarantee that you will become a non-smoker.

If you don't become a non-smoker it will simply be because you did not follow the instructions in this book *to the letter*. It is of the utmost importance that you understand this "following instructions to the letter" concept; otherwise you will be giving your denial mechanism a foothold. If you *do* give it a foothold, you can be damned sure that sooner or later it will have you smoking again! So once again – if you want to stop smoking be sure to follow the instructions.

The following chapter will help you to understand nicotine addiction and will go some way towards explaining why you continue to smoke, even though deep down you don't really want to!

CHAPTER 1 - UNDERSTANDING ADDICTION

The first thing you need to do is to establish beyond any reasonable doubt that you are, in fact, a nicotine addict.

You may feel uncomfortable with this idea - most people do not like to think of themselves as any kind of addict because the word 'addict' is commonly associated with images of drugs, junkies, squalor and all sorts of seediness. More importantly for our purposes, addiction of any sort is generally (and wrongly) regarded as a weakness.

Some people think that to admit to addiction is an admission of personal inadequacy, and there are also (believe it or not) some individuals who think that addiction of any sort is a moral failure, and that in general, addicts are 'bad' people!

Let's get this clear. There is nothing morally wrong with being addicted to nicotine; or anything else for that matter. Nor is addiction a 'weakness'. Those who try to perpetuate these attitudes are not being realistic about the whole realm of addiction within our society today. Addiction of all kinds is rampant and the vast majority of individuals are addicted to one substance / behavior or another.

Take nicotine for example, roughly 30 percent of the adult population in most western countries are addicted to it. If you then add the number of people addicted to caffeine in tea, coffee, cola drinks and chocolate, and further add the number of people addicted to alcohol and street or prescription drugs, then you are looking at a populace with a *minority* of non addicts.

This is especially true if you include all the other mostly unseen addictions such as exercise, sex, work or computer games. The point being is that to admit to being a nicotine addict is simply to identify your addiction as nicotine, as opposed to any of these other addictions. There is no shame or weakness in being addicted to nicotine and admission as such is just recognition of the facts.

Why is it important to admit to being addicted?

ADMISSION OF ADDICTION IS OF <u>FUNDAMENTAL IMPORTANCE</u> IN THE BATTLE TO BECOME NICOTINE FREE!

One of the psychological 'defenses' that goes hand in hand with all addictions is the process of denial.

IF YOU ARE A NICOTINE ADDICT (and if you are a regular smoker you almost certainly are) *THEN YOU WILL BE AFFECTED BY THE PROCESS OF DENIAL.*

There are no words that can adequately express the importance of that last statement. In fact it is so important to understand that I am going to say it again: **IF YOU ARE A NICOTINE ADDICT THEN <u>YOU WILL</u> BE AFFECTED BY THE PROCESS OF DENIAL!**

What is denial?

Denial is the method adopted by your unconscious mind to keep you feeding nicotine to your body. The easiest way to understand why on earth your own mind is attempting to get you to poison yourself with nicotine is to think of it in these terms:

One of the functions of your unconscious mind is to ensure that you go through life feeling as little discomfort as possible, irrespective of how it manages to achieve this. Unfortunately, your unconscious mind does not make value judgments. It doesn't, for instance, say to itself "Mmm.., I've stopped smoking and I'm starting to feel uncomfortable, I would like a smoke, but I don't want to risk cancer so I will just tolerate the withdrawal symptoms until they go away."

If your unconscious was able to make value judgments of this kind - ie., I won't do (a) because it will result in (b), then no one would have any real difficulty in giving up. When this situation arises, i.e., when you start to feel the symptoms of nicotine withdrawal, this is what you can expect from the treacherous little 'voice' that is your unconscious:

Firstly, your unconscious will notice your discomfort. It will then compare your feelings of discomfort to the memory bank of feelings stored in your mind, and will decide on what it believes to be the source of your discomfort. In no time at all it will figure out that the last time you felt these negative feelings you were able to relieve them by having a cigarette.

Having found the simple solution to your problems, it will send a message to your conscious mind. That message is likely to be "Have a smoke". The problem now lies with the conflict that arises between your conscious and unconscious mind. By the time you get to the stage of feeling withdrawal, you have already consciously made the decision that you are never going to smoke again. This is when the real battle begins. Before we look at this whole battle process, let me tell you some more about this destructive unconscious 'voice'. This 'voice' is generally stronger and more determined than your conscious mind - a *lot* stronger and a *lot* more determined. For this reason **when** you first hear this 'voice' telling you to smoke, you will need to immediately be on your guard. Here's why:

When you first stop smoking your conscious mind will start of with a high level of motivation to carry through your resolve not to smoke. Now, all would be well if your little 'voice' was to agree with your decision to stop, and think: "Fair enough, I'll just not smoke."

However, let me assure you that is never, ever, going to happen. Like a spoilt brat, this little 'voice' will then resort to all sorts of mental trickery in order that you feed it the nicotine that it so desperately wants. In fact, it will resort to levels of deception so low and cunning, that at first you will hardly believe it possible. Here is a typical conscious / unconscious dialogue:

U: = Unconscious   **C:** = Conscious

C: "Oh, oh, I am starting to feel cravings"

U: "I'll have a smoke"

C: "No I have stopped, I must be strong" (Your unconscious may then wait until the craving becomes a bit stronger then:)

U: "I'll have a smoke now, I can stop again tomorrow."

C: "No, I mustn't, I haven't really given it a proper go." (Your unconscious might then wait until you are a bit more vulnerable, say a few hours later when you have just had a cup of tea and you are really gasping for a smoke, then:)

U: "I'll just have this one cigarette with my tea, I never really had a proper 'last' cigarette."

Some people may relapse at this stage and will decide to smoke. For those with stronger resolve the conversation may continue along these lines:

C: "No, I will try to stick it out a bit longer." (Your unconscious may wait until you are more vulnerable, say maybe two days later when perhaps the cravings feel quite intense)

U: "Huh, they told me that this would get easier but it's getting harder; sod the lot of them, I am going to have a smoke."

C: "No, wait a minute, I really do have to give it my best shot, I'll get through this bad patch soon enough." (Your unconscious may then do one of several things. For instance it may allow you to feel almost no negative feelings for a couple of days and then when you are feeling good about how strong you have been and how easy' it has been, feed you with this almost classic line:)

U: "See, I knew that I could give up smoking easily, in fact it was so easy I am pretty sure I could have a smoke now and stop again with no bother. Yeah, I think I'll celebrate with a final cigarette." (You would be shocked by the number of people who have been suckered by that line!)

If, by this stage, you still have not succumbed to the little 'voice' then it will simply become even more devious. Remember, the sole purpose in life of this little 'voice' is to get you to smoke and it has no qualms about how it achieves this goal.

The next trick up its sleeve will probably be to convince your conscious mind that the pain of withdrawal is actually much worse than it really is. (You will be looking at this pain issue in some depth in the next section.) Your unconscious will also try to confuse you by allowing the feelings of both tiredness and hunger to masquerade as withdrawal:

U: (After a long and tiring day) "I'm absolutely exhausted and I'm gasping, I'm going to have a smoke, I'll stop again at the beginning of the month when my work schedule isn't as hectic."

Again, many people will drop out at this (or a similar) point.

On and on this little 'voice' goes, relentlessly pursuing its perverted goal. In reality, it is actually even worse than I can describe here because its repertoire of excuses or justifications is almost infinite. If all the above fails to achieve its aim, then it can resort to tactics such as attributing just about anything negative that happens to you, to giving up smoking.

Say, for example, that you are a salesperson. You have been off cigarettes for three days and you have had a bad day selling. The little 'voice' in your head starts to tell you that "I just can't sell as well when I don't have my cigarettes to help me concentrate."

Now, you may think this believable, until you consider that there is normally a bad day or two every week, irrespective of whether you smoke or not. The reality is that this may well be just one of those days - nothing at all to do with whether or not you have smoked! Again, it is just this little 'voice' in full trickery mode.

Another way the 'voice' operates is to have you constantly focus on your pain. Say, for example you develop a headache. The little 'voice' will get you to focus on it to such an extent that you will believe that it is the worst headache of your life and that the only thing that will get rid of it will be to have a smoke. Again, it is simply an illusion created by your unconscious, in order to get you to smoke.

Given the deviousness and subtlety of your little 'voice', you will need to learn how to become aware of the true level of any pain you might feel (mental or physical), how to recognize and respond to its manipulations, and how to say "no" to its thousand and one reasons for why you should smoke again.

You will learn how to do this a little further on, but first, let's go back to the big question!

ARE YOU A NICOTINE ADDICT?

In order to answer this question we first of all need to establish a definition for addiction. Before we look at this definition I would ask you to try and empty your mind of any preconceived notions that you may have of addiction, and to come to this question with an open mind.

As part of an assignment I was writing many years ago at university, I had to study several definitions of addiction and to finally settle on the one that would be the most useful to use as a model for actually working with addicts. The definition that I finally settled on is the one used by the World Health Organization. It states (simplified) that an addict is anyone who suffers physical and / or psychological negative effects when the substance they are using is withdrawn, to the extent where they would feel relief if given more of the substance.

If we are to use this definition here then it should be easy enough to establish whether or not you are a nicotine addict.

What follows is a simple questionnaire which you need to answer as honestly as possible with either a yes or a no:

1. HAVE YOU EVER TRIED TO STOP BEFORE AND FAILED?

2. HAVE YOU EVER FELT PANICKY WHEN YOU COULDN'T GET A CIGARETTE?

3. HAVE YOU EVER FELT NICOTINE WITHDRAWAL SYMPTOMS?

4. HAVE YOU EVER USED CIGARETTES TO CALM YOUR NERVES IN A CRISIS?

5. HAVE YOU EVER FELT RELIEF ON LIGHTING UP A CIGARETTE?

6. HAVE YOU EVER HAD A CIGARETTE IMMEDIATELY AFTER GETTING OUT OF BED IN THE MORNING?

7. HAVE YOU EVER SAID THAT YOU WERE ADDICTED TO SMOKING?

8. DO YOU USUALLY EAT A LOT MORE WHEN YOU QUIT SMOKING?

9. DO YOU EXPERIENCE A FEELING OF 'HOLLOWNESS' IN YOUR CHEST IF YOU HAVEN'T SMOKED FOR A WHILE?

10. DOES THE THOUGHT OF STOPPING SMOKING SOMETIMES SCARE YOU?

11.   DO YOU EVER DOUBT YOUR ABILITY TO STAY STOPPED?

12.   HAVE YOU EVER STOPPED BEFORE, ONLY TO LET THAT LITTLE 'VOICE' TALK YOU INTO SMOKING AGAIN?

13.   DO YOU FEEL BAD ABOUT BEING A SMOKER?

14.   DO YOU EVER SMOKE TO HELP YOU CONCENTRATE?

15.   HAVE YOU EVER USED HELP TO TRY AND STOP SMOKING? (Hypnotism, books, nicotine gum, patches etc.)

Now count the total number of times you answered yes.

Finished? Ok then, now, I'm not going to tell you that if you answered "yes" to so many questions then you are a nicotine addict and if you answered "no" to so many then you are not.

This questionnaire is designed to be an *awareness* exercise to enable you to realize (if you don't already) that you are an addict. To illustrate this point, take question 15 alone - who other than someone who had a real problem stopping would need to buy a book to help them? In fact, who would answer yes to even one of these questions if they didn't fall into the category nicotine addict'?

You made an unconscious admission of your addiction as soon as you decided to try this book. In practical terms, the more of these questions you answered "yes" to, the stronger and more ingrained your nicotine addiction is likely to be. This next declaration is important. It is where you are going to acknowledge to yourself that you are an addict and that you are going to stop smoking.

When you can agree that you are an addict and that you are going to stop, then immediately sign the following declaration and move on to the next section. If you still have difficulty with the concept of being an addict then take the time to re-read the previous questionnaire and related matter, and consider your own case in considerable detail, and with an open mind.

It is important for you to see that using the above definition you really are addicted to nicotine and that an admission as such will close one of the doors that could well lead to your failure when the going gets a bit tough.

If you don't admit to your addiction you may find it all too easy to start smoking again. Sooner or later, through your little 'voice', you will tell yourself that you don't *really* have a problem and, therefore, you can smoke now because you could easily stop any time you wanted to! Be aware that if you have told yourself this in the past, it hasn't worked, because you are reading this book and must (presumably) still be a smoker!

Denial of your addiction is exactly what your little 'voice' wants and denial is simply setting yourself up for failure!

DECLARATION:

Congratulations! Now that you have admitted that you are a nicotine addict, you are on the road to becoming an ex smoker, but there are a couple of things more that you need to know about the nature of your addiction:

NO MATTER WHAT YOU DO YOU WILL ALWAYS BE A NICOTINE ADDICT

This may sound like an odd thing to be telling you in a book about overcoming addiction. However, it is of the utmost importance that you understand this concept otherwise relapse is waiting for you just around the corner.

Once you have acquired an addiction you cannot be cured of it. Two years from now, say, even if you have been totally smoke free for the whole two years, you might decide to have a smoke. Just the one of course, (yes its that little 'voice' again!) to celebrate say perhaps, the birth of your son. As soon as nicotine enters your body the whole addiction process which you have managed to put to sleep for two years, is suddenly reactivated.

On finishing that cigarette you will find that two hours later you feel like having another one. Now the little 'voice' that had been lying more or less dormant for the last two years, save for a few token appearances at vulnerable or celebratory times, suddenly shakes itself awake, and in no time at all is going at full strength. The conscious / unconscious dialogue begins all over again:

U: "Well, I know I said I'd only have the one but it's a really special occasion. I'll smoke up until midnight tonight and then I'll stop again."

Yeah, right! This could happen after twenty, or forty years never mind two!

So what is the solution?

Well actually the solution is quite simple. Within the first month or two after stopping, you will notice your little 'voice' has begun to quiet down. With every passing day the 'voice' will become not only less frequent, but also less intense. After these first couple of months, staying stopped will no longer be a problem that you need to make an strenuous effort to overcome, except, perhaps for the very odd occasion when you are feeling particularly tired, hungry, angry, happy, lonely, stressed or otherwise vulnerable. Even then the 'voice' will probably only make a small token appearance, but only

PROVIDED THAT YOU DO NOT UNDER ANY CIRCUMSTANCES ALLOW YOUR BODY TO INGEST NICOTINE.

Or, to put it another way, provided that you do not smoke. Not ever, not 'just this one', not a pipe, or a cigar, or a 'joint', or even a single draw of a low tar cigarette.

If nicotine gets into your system *at all*, you may well be heading straight back to square one. I realize that this sounds terribly daunting and may make you feel that you are about to engage in a lifelong and difficult battle. In one sense you *are* going to be engaged in this battle for life, because as I mentioned earlier, there is no permanent cure for nicotine addiction.

However, you can rest easy, because after you have succeeded in your initial battle with your little 'voice', and it becomes dormant, you will never really have any difficulty staying stopped. The worst you can expect is the occasional light pang, provided of course that you do not put any nicotine into your body in any shape or form.

Before we move on to the next section, let's take a brief look at what you have covered so far:

First of all you learned that most people suffer from one form of addiction or another and that there is no shame or weakness in being addicted to nicotine.

You learned that denial is an integral part of your addiction and that it involves your unconscious mind trying to get you to smoke, in order that you don't feel the pain of withdrawal.

You also discovered that your denial doesn't care about how it achieves its aim, and that it will create and feed invalid excuses to your conscious mind.

You admitted that you were an addict and signed a declaration to that effect, and you agreed to stop smoking when you finish this book. You learned that you will always be an addict but that after a couple of months your addiction will cause you little or no problem, provided that you never let nicotine get into your body.

In the next chapter you are going to be looking at pain, and how your little 'voice' will be using pain as its primary weapon!

CHAPTER 2 - DEALING WITH PAIN

When I use the word pain in this book I am referring not just to physical pain, ie., the type that makes you go "ow", but also to psychological pain. Pain that includes anger, jealousy, grief, despair, loneliness, guilt, resentment, fear, sadness, depression and hate.

These forms of emotional pain are the ones most likely to weaken your initial resolve to stop smoking and create for you, through that little 'voice', the excuse you need (or more accurately, want) to start smoking again.

Why do you need to examine pain?

The answer to this question is that each of us has a pain threshold that is unique to ourselves. This threshold is partly established at birth and partly acquired by our experiences as we go through life. Once this threshold has been exceeded, we will allow ourselves to operate outside the normal boundaries of our personalities.

For example, most of us have at some time or another promised to keep a secret and have been strong in our resolve. Had this resolve been threatened by physical or emotional pain however, it may soon have crumbled. The likelihood of you keeping a secret will always be in direct relation to the amount of pain that you have to endure.

If you were being asked to tell your secret by someone who was giving you gentle slaps on the back of your hand for a period of ten minutes, you would probably have little or   no difficulty in keeping quiet.

If, however, you were being burnt at regular intervals with red hot pokers over a period of weeks, it is extremely likely that you would tell your torturers whatever they wanted to know, (and probably a whole lot more!) and to hell with your original resolve!

An extreme example, granted, but it does clearly illustrate the link between pain, and failure to keep a resolution. If you view this pain / failure link in the context of stopping smoking, then it becomes clear that in order to increase your chances of staying stopped, you will need to look at how you can reduce all the areas of pain and potential pain in your life.

Let's start now by taking a look at pain itself. Pain is one of the areas in your life where your little 'voice' has a lot of control and when you stop smoking your little 'voice' will steer you towards focusing on any emotional or physical pain that you might have.

It will try to convince you that this pain is almost unbearable and of course that the pain is there because you are not smoking and therefore you should have a smoke! (Just the one of course!)

Back in the land of reality it transpires that almost every day brings some level of emotional or physical pain for most people. Perhaps in the form of a headache, or a row at the office, or a final demand from the gas board. Perhaps a disagreement with your mother, or a touch of arthritis, or a bad cold. Maybe a sleepless night or a pulled muscle. It could be an embarrassing Freudian slip, or a wasp sting or, a bad report from your daughters school. Perhaps a whisper about job losses at your factory, or a missed promotion - and so on and so on.

This list is but a very small sample of all the potential areas for pain in your life and it could be extended almost indefinitely. It is sad but unfortunately true, that for most of us, a lot of the time, life can be quite painful in one way or another.

Stopping smoking will not make life any tougher, but at the start it will make you feel a little more vulnerable. This in turn will make you suddenly focus on all this negative everyday pain. Once again your little 'voice' will step in and it will try to tell you that life wasn't this tough before you stopped smoking. Of course it was - most of the time you simply didn't notice!

Now then, how can all this information can be of use to you?

If you become aware of the fact that you are going to be feeling a little vulnerable for a short period of time, then you are going to be in a much better position to be able to deal effectively with any pain that comes your way without having to resort to smoking.

Let's look again at one of the prices that you earlier agreed to pay:

You said that you were prepared to feel at least some pain. That's good because when you start to feel some withdrawal discomfort, (which you will you do not have to panic, get things out of perspective, and end up smoking You can simply monitor your discomfort and tell yourself that:

THIS DISCOMFORT IS THE PRICE I HAVE AGREED TO PAY TO BECOME A NON SMOKER.

Once you have agreed that you are prepared to tolerate a little discomfort, you will find that you can effectively manage this discomfort by using the techniques put forward later on in this book. You can further lessen your pain by learning to view it from outside the context of that little 'voice'. That 'voice' will be telling you all the time that your discomfort is unbearable and that you would be better off smoking.

The pain however, is not at all unbearable, but for the most part it is an illusion created by the little 'voice' of your unconscious. You can actually measure your discomfort by comparing your feelings to a simple pain strength table.

Before using the following table, complete a head to toe scan of yourself in order to monitor how much pain you are in. Here's how to do it. When you first feel the pangs of withdrawal ask yourself what *exactly* it is that you are feeling.

The following is a list of commonly reported symptoms of nicotine withdrawal and it is very likely that your symptoms will be amongst them.

- A FEELING OF 'EMPTINESS' IN THE CHEST

- A FEELING OF HUNGER

- A FEELING OF TIREDNESS

- A HEADACHE

- A DRY MOUTH

- A CONFUSED FEELING

- A TENDENCY TOWARDS IRRITABILITY

- A FEELING OF HELPLESSNESS OR WEAKNESS

These symptoms make up the bulk of the feelings you may experience as part of your withdrawal. In addition, because we are all so unique in our physical and psychological construction, you may of course feel symptoms other than those mentioned here.

Also, because of our uniqueness these symptoms will be felt by each person to a different degree, so if you happen to be one of the lucky ones, they may present you with absolutely no difficulty at all. However, if you are like most people you will probably feel one or more of these symptoms and when you do, you can compare each one to the following scale:

1. NO PAIN AT ALL

2. ALMOST NO PAIN

3. A LITTLE PAIN

4. PAINFUL

5. VERY PAINFUL

6. EXTREMELY PAINFUL

7. ABSOLUTELY UNBEARABLE

Here's how to use the body check and pain strength table:

Say for example that you stopped smoking two hours ago and you begin to feel the symptoms of nicotine withdrawal. What should you do?

The first thing you need to do is to complete the head to toe body check to see exactly where the problem lies. A typical body check would be something like this:

HEAD   -   A bit sore.

NECK   -   OK.

ARMS   -   OK.

CHEST   -   A very empty, hollow sort of feeling.

ABDOMEN -   A kind of hungry feeling.

LEGS   -   A tired feeling and a bit shaky

FEET   -   OK.

MENTAL STATE -   A bit confused and a bit angry, feeling a little panicky.

Now, what you need to do is to take each symptom separately and compare it to the pain strength table. I can absolutely guarantee that once you think **honestly** about it, you will be surprised at just how low you register each symptom on this table. For instance, one of the most common withdrawal symptoms that leads to failure is that feeling of 'emptiness' in the chest.

If you are unaware of the tricks of your little 'voice' and have not thought consciously about just how bad this discomfort really is, then in no time at all you can lose the true perspective, start to believe that you are in agony, and throw in the towel. If, however, you do have an awareness of this little 'voice's' tendency to make you focus on your symptoms, and you look at your pain realistically, (by means of the body scan and pain chart) you will soon discover that the pain really is for the most part an illusion.

You may well find that what at first appears to be a vast, unbearable emptiness raging within your lungs, when critically examined, turns out in fact to be nothing more unpleasant than a feeling similar to hunger, or, perhaps, like a slight pressure on your sternum. This illusory effect applies to **all** of your symptoms and all you need to do to overcome this illusion is to think about each symptom as it occurs, and measure it on the pain chart in order to see it for what it *really* is.

If you do this exercise as honestly as possible, you will find that you rarely encounter a pain or discomfort that registers above 'a bit painful'.

If this turns out to be your experience, as is likely, then you will be depriving your little 'voice' of the central focus of its power. That is, the illusion that you are in so much discomfort that you should start smoking again. If, however, you are one of the few individuals who have an exceptionally low tolerance for discomfort, (and of course your little 'voice' will no doubt try to convince you that you have the lowest pain threshold of anyone who ever lived!) then fear not, for all is not lost!

If you discover in assessing your pain honestly, that you are continually registering in the very painful or unbearable areas of the pain level chart, then you still have a few options open to you. First of all it is important to know this:

NICOTINE CRAVING COMES IN BURSTS OF THREE TO FIVE MINUTES.

Now, I don't care how unbearable you think your cravings are because there is almost no one who, if they are serious about stopping smoking, cannot tolerate three to five minutes of pain or discomfort at a time. Let's face it, we are not talking about being run through with flaming swords, we are talking primarily about feeling 'empty' or 'hungry' or having a bit of a headache.

Furthermore, not only do the cravings come in bursts of three to five minutes, but as time wears on these attacks become less and less frequent and also less intense. What this means to you is that if you can get over the first few days, your task will become progressively easier.

Remember that it is not going to be a totally pain free ride, but you have agreed to pay the price of at least some pain!

Finally, in this section here is some further advice for those who need even more assistance to deal with these early stages of withdrawal.

Keep in your mind the following saying for when the going gets rough. It is a saying used by recovering addicts and alcoholics all over the world, when they feel that they are starting to waver. The saying is simply this:

"THIS TOO, SHALL PASS"

You will find that the bad times *always pass*. You also now know that it is not always going to be tough, just every now and again and for short periods. Always remember that after the first few days, with each passing hour, you are getting further and further away from your addiction and its symptoms, and continually closer to being a symptom free non smoker.

The final tool to be discussed here is also one used by recovering addicts and alcoholics the world over. They use this when they find staying abstinent difficult . It is an expression that most of you will have heard before and it is this: **"ONE DAY AT A TIME"**

This method has proved its worth time and time again and it works like this:

When you feel yourself starting to struggle and your little 'voice' seems to be operating on overdrive, tell yourself that:

"NO MATTER WHAT HAPPENS I WILL NOT SMOKE FOR 24 HOURS"

At first glance this might seem like a license to smoke *after* twenty four hours, but of course it doesn't quite work like that. First of all, after twenty four hours you may not be in such a negative mood, or you may no longer be feeling any withdrawal symptoms and, therefore, might not want to smoke.

Furthermore, all you have to do at the end of twenty four hours is to make another resolution not to smoke for the next twenty four hours. At first glance this may seem to be a bit daft, but on closer examination it makes a lot of sense.

Many of us could tolerate things for twenty four hours that would seem impossible to consider for a lifetime. If you put yourself in the position where no matter what happens you will not smoke for the next twenty four hours, then soon enough you will have strung together enough days to take you far enough away from your Withdrawal to allow you to succeed.

OK, let's now take a quick look at what you have learned in this chapter:

✓ First of all, you learned that there are different types of pain and that each of us has a different pain threshold.

✓ You then explored the link between excessive pain and starting smoking again, and how that little 'voice' will try to force you to focus intensely on everyday pain, with a view to weakening you to the point of smoking.

✓ Next, you were reminded that you had agreed to tolerate at least a little discomfort in the short term and how to actually lessen any discomfort by getting things into perspective.

✓ You were shown how to do this by completing a simple body scan, and comparing your symptoms to a pain level chart, where you discovered that your pain is nowhere near as severe as you first thought.

✓ If you discovered that you still couldn't tolerate the discomfort, you then learned that the actual cravings only ever became really intense for periods of between three and five minutes, and that you could deal with this inconvenience by the knowledge that it would soon pass, because it always does.

✓ You also learned that you could tolerate the milder cravings which are often present by agreeing to accept them as part of the price for becoming a non smoker and by living 'just for today.'

CHAPTER 3 - DEALING WITH YOUR UNCONSCIOUS

In this chapter you are going to continue looking at the little 'voice' and some of its more common tactics and learn how you can be ready to take control when it tries to convince you that you need to smoke.

What you are going to do now is to look in some depth at the little 'voice' and prepare yourself for the battle that will begin within a couple of hours of stopping smoking. Actually, your little 'voice' will **now know** of your intentions to stop smoking and will already be trying to put obstacles in your way!

You may, for instance, have had thoughts while reading this book along the lines of "I'll read this book now, but I won't stop until the end of the month in order that the information can sink in." Or perhaps "Oh dear, I don't like the thought of all this self-analysis stuff, perhaps I should just try nicotine patches instead. Yeah, that's it, I'll buy a supply at the end of the month."

Again, if you listen to this little 'voice' you are doomed to failure. The only realistic way of stopping smoking is to put this little 'voice' in its place by agreeing to pay the price of some discomfort, making a resolution to stop smoking straight away, stopping, and finally, staying stopped, no matter what happens.

Here is an analogy from my own life that helps to illustrate the effectiveness of carrying on with a resolution in spite of feeling discomfort: When I was running a charity in Belfast for recovering addicts, we regularly entered the Belfast / Dublin Maracycle, a two hundred mile cycle over two days.

At the forty mile point in this cycle there is a mountain to cross, and one stretch of road by the name of Newry Hill, is very steep and climbs for about two miles. Each of the first three years that I'd participated, I had simply cycled about a quarter of the way up this hill, got off my bike and walked up the rest. On the fourth year my good friend Arty Magill called me aside at the start of the Maracycle and said to me:

"I know how you can get up Newry Hill!"

" Oh really?" I replied with more than a modicum of disbelief. "Yes," he replied "When you reach the bottom of the hill, keep pedaling and no matter what happens, don't stop until you get to the top."

Now as you might imagine I was, at first, none too impressed with this pearl of wisdom. However, when I actually took the time to think clearly about what he meant, I discovered that his advice was pretty much faultless.

Cycling that hill was certainly well within my physical capability because, although I was not particularly fit, I was a young and reasonably strong man and, in the previous years, I had observed the majority of participants successfully tackle this hill, and this included many pensioners!

When I thought about this a bit more I realized that the real problem was that on previous occasions I had used my discomfort (tired legs, a bright red face and panting lungs) as an excuse to stop and walk.

In brief, I had not agreed to pay the price of some discomfort to achieve this goal, so when the chips where down I simply gave up. On this forth occasion, however after Artys' little chat, I decided that when I reached Newry Hill I *would* pay the price and keep pedaling no matter what.

What actually happened was that I cycled up that hill with no real difficulty at all. In fact I stood on the pedals and sprinted the second half of it, having realized that it was nowhere near as bad as I had let it become in my imagination.

This simple advice turned my whole experience of this hill around. I have since adapted it to many situations where I knew for certain that if I determinedly and resolutely followed one specific course of action then it would end with a specific result.

You could, in fact, use this simple method alone to stop smoking; after all, you know for certain that if you don't smoke a cigarette, no matter how uncomfortable you feel, then eventually all your withdrawal symptoms would disappear and sooner or later you would become a symptom free nonsmoker.

This is exactly the course of action that you *will* be following, except you will be equipped with all the tools you will need to help make your journey a much more tolerable and comfortable one!

Right, now back to the little 'voice':

The first thing you need to know is that this 'voice' is not going to sound any different to you than your normal everyday thoughts. That being the case, how then can you tell if it is your conscious or unconscious mind that is producing your thoughts? Well, the answer is quite simple.

You made a conscious decision to stop smoking. There is never, ever, going to be a valid reason to reverse this decision, therefore, any thoughts that you have in relation to smoking again must be ones deliberately generated by your unconscious in the form of the little 'voice', in order that you may avoid feeling pain or discomfort. So, all you have to do is to notice if you are making any excuse at all to start smoking again and, if you are, you can be sure it is your little 'voice' that is responsible. Simple eh?

I would like you to look at the list below of some of the more common justifications for starting smoking again, many of which you may well experience. I will also give you examples of how to answer these negative thoughts, and with a little practice you will find that recognizing and dealing with this little 'voice' can become quite easy. These are some of the most commonly experienced thoughts that can lead to relapse:

1. **"I'll just have this one and then I'll stop again."**

This is by far the most often used excuse in order to alleviate the discomfort of withdrawal. Unfortunately, it almost always results in the permanent resumption of smoking because once nicotine has been reintroduced to your system; it is like starting back at square one again. The cravings after this one cigarette will return to being as strong as when you first stopped smoking, and the little 'voice' will have all of its original determination.

In this situation it is all too easy to delude yourself into agreeing that you may as well be hung for a sheep as for a lamb. Even this process of failure is usually split into stages in order to lessen the blow to your ego. For example, you may start by telling yourself that you will "just have the one smoke" and then you may change that to "just smoking for the rest of the day" and then "until the end of the week", by which time of course you will have little or no resolve left at all. No, the only way to avoid this trap is this:

DON'T SMOKE A SINGLE CIGARETTE.

Or even one drag of a cigarette, for any reason at all.

So, when you hear this little 'voice' telling you to "take just one", (and believe me, you will) have your reply ready "No - it is not worth it, it will almost certainly lead to my failure."

2. **"I feel like I am going to pieces, I will stop some other time."**

This, too, is a common 'justification' and leads to the failure of many. First of all, stopping at "some other time" is likely to feel just as uncomfortable as it does now, and, therefore, you are simply deluding yourself in order to avoid this present discomfort. Secondly, it is highly unlikely that you will "fall to pieces" and it is very likely that if you sit tight through this period you will find that it will pass quite quickly - remember the saying used by addicts the world over: **"This too, shall pass."**

Finally, remember that you did agree to pay the price of some discomfort in order to achieve your goal of becoming a non smoker. This short term discomfort is in reality, a very small price to pay.

When you hear your 'little voice' telling you that you are falling apart and that you will stop some other time reply: *"There is no other time that will be better than now. I am simply going through a temporary rough patch, and it will pass"*

3. "I have had a terrible day at work, I will have a smoke."

No matter how bad things were at work smoking is never going to make them any better. You already know that whether or not you are a smoker you are always going to encounter some bad days - that's life, and there is simply no avoiding this fact.

It is unrealistic to imagine that taking a cigarette will change anything, other than changing you from being a successful non smoker into a smoking failure. When you hear the little voice telling you that you deserve a smoke after such a hard day, reply:

"No, I know that life is sometimes hard and this is just one of those days. I will not smoke because smoking will not solve anything and, in fact, it will probably make me feel like a failure. This day is OK, because no matter what else has happened, I haven't smoked and that makes me both strong and successful."

4. "I am angry and I am taking it out on my kids and husband, they don't deserve this. I am going to smoke.

What they really don't deserve is to be visiting you in hospital, dying from some smoking related illness. They don't deserve to be subjected to passive smoking and your children don't deserve to be given the role model that smoking is OK. If your concern is really for your family then the fact that they might have to tolerate you being grumpy for a short while is of little consequence. When you hear the little voice telling you that your family are suffering, reply:

"This is a short term situation, they will suffer far more in the long run if I start smoking again."

5. **"I am putting on too much weight. If I start smoking again my weight will return to normal."**

Because this is an excuse frequently used by people to start smoking again (particularly women) the next section of this book concentrates on stopping smoking without gaining weight. There is no reason at all to gain weight if you do not want to.

Even if you do not follow the advice for maintaining your current weight, you will probably find that any weight gain is temporary and that after a few months your weight will return to normal. As compared to the benefits of stopping smoking, this whole business of potential weight gain should be regarded as a fairly minor and totally manageable affair.

When you hear the little 'voice' telling you that smoking is the solution to any weight gain reply:

"No, this weight gain is temporary and I can avoid weight gain by following the advice given in this book."

6. "I'll only smoke when I'm out in the pub with my friends."

This is an area where you need to be particularly on your guard.

Once you have consumed even a little alcohol your original resolve will be reduced enormously and the little 'voice' will immediately take advantage of your weakened condition.

Many, many, ex-smokers start smoking again when they go to the pub, or take a few drinks at home. There is also a direct correlation between how much you drink and how likely you are to start smoking again - the more drinks the greater the risk of relapse. It is very important to emphasize here the link between drinking alcohol and resuming smoking.

Every time you go to the pub or take a few drinks you are putting yourself in a potential relapse situation. There are, of course, things that you can do in order to reduce this risk. You could simply stop drinking for as long as it takes for you to be certain that you are not at risk of smoking again.

So strong is the link between drinking alcohol and smoking that temporary total abstinence is the course of action that I recommend. However, I do realize that this might, for some of you, seem like a mammoth task to undertake in addition to not smoking. So if you feel that you really do have to drink or go to pubs, there are still things that you can do in order to minimize the risk of starting smoking again:

✓ You could stay of alcohol for the first two weeks.

✓ You could drink less frequently than normal.

✓ You could go to the pub and drink soft drinks for a few weeks.

✓ You could drink less alcohol each time you go out. (Or in the home.)

✓ You could ask your social partners to encourage you not to smoke when you are out.

✓ You could ask your partner or a good friend to phone you when you are out to check on your progress and offer you support.

Remember, all of these actions are temporary. Soon enough, usually within a couple of months, you will be strong enough to handle most situations without this high level of support, and without smoking.

So, if your little 'voice' tells you to smoke when you are socializing with a few drinks, reply:

"No, I don't need to smoke in order to socialize and if I don't smoke now, then soon enough I won't miss smoking at all."

7. **"Oh, I don't give a damn; I am going to smoke and to hell with the consequences."**

Perhaps this little tactic should have been mentioned at the very beginning of this list. Without doubt it is the one thought that sooner or later you are going to encounter. This is the most powerful of all the weapons in your little 'voice's' armory.

Your unconscious knows that if you start to think about whether or not you should smoke, (particularly now that you are now in possession of all the information in this book) then you are almost certainly going to come to the decision to stick it out and not smoke.

So what does your little 'voice' do then?

Easy - if your new found knowledge leads you to decide not to smoke then your unconscious tricks you into not accessing this knowledge. You are told by it to disregard everything you know in order that you make a bad decision - a decision based not at all on logic but purely on feeling.

Simplified, it goes like this:

" I am in pain, a smoke will take away my pain, don't think about anything else, just take a smoke."

This tactic is a real killer and you need to be particularly aware of it in order to stand a good chance of defeating it. When you hear your mind thinking anything along the "I don't care" lines, be ready to respond.

Tell yourself:

"I might not feel like I care right now, but this is a temporary feeling. Smoking now would ruin everything. I realize that the little 'voice' is trying to get me and I will not give in to it!"

There are going to be many situations where your little 'voice' will try to get to you, and the real secret of defeating it is to regard it as your worst enemy.

Approach this whole affair as though it is a personal battle between you and this little 'voice', and that your life depends on you defeating it. The reality is that in many ways your life *does* depend on you succeeding. You may find it extremely helpful to think of this little voice as someone you know and who you really don't like. Imagine that every time you hear it trying to get you to smoke, it is that person you dislike, trying to get the better of you.

It also helps to congratulate yourself each time that you recognize and defeat this 'voice'. Put a piece of paper on a convenient wall and a little tick on it each time you win a battle with this 'voice'. You will then be able to see just how often it raises its ugly head. This little 'voice' can become easy to defeat with practice, once, that is, you become aware of it, and are determined not to let it sucker you into smoking.

✓ You have now reached a point of understanding where you are nearly ready to begin this whole battle process with your unconscious.

✓ You have become aware of the fact that you are a nicotine addict and that not feeding your addiction causes you discomfort.

✓ You have learned that your unconscious will try all sorts of tricks in order to get you to ease this discomfort by smoking. These tricks include feeding your conscious mind excuses and getting you to focus on your pain in order that you come to believe that it is more intense than it actually is.

✓ You have learned how to tell the difference between your conscious and unconscious 'voices' and how to analyse your pain in order to put it into perspective.

✓ You have also learned that heavy withdrawal never lasts more than a few minutes at a time and you now know that these rough patches always pass. If you happen to be particularly sensitive to discomfort, then you now know that you can live 'one day at a time' or even one hour at a time if needs be.

✓ You are also aware that there is never any valid reason for smoking again and that there are going to be times when you are particularly vulnerable.

All you need to do now is to set up a suitable support structure and you will be ready to begin stopping.

The next chapter will deal with this support issue and show you what you need to do in order to build up enough support to allow you to succeed.

CHAPTER 4 - CREATING SUPPORT STRUCTURES

This next statement is of fundamental importance:

YOU WILL STAND A MUCH GREATER CHANCE OF SUCCEEDING IF YOU USE ALL OF THE FOLLOWING SUPPORT STRATEGIES!

Using support has always been a stumbling block for people trying to tackle their addictions. Addicts, by their very nature, have a strong Tendency to resist support and I have lost count of the times that I have seen addicts relapse because of their reluctance to utilize available assistance. Curious indeed, when you consider that this reluctance sometimes can cost addicts their lives.

There are several reasons why an addict may refuse to use support and it is important that you look at Some of these reasons here. If you are one of those people who cringe at the thought of asking for help, you may benefit from exploring the reasons behind your reluctance. Receiving adequate support will in many cases mean the difference between success and failure.

Probably the most common reason for not asking for support is this:

YOU DO NOT WANT TO APPEAR WEAK

Western society has a tendency to socialize its citizens into believing that it is wrong to ask for help, and fosters the belief that individuals should be able to manage on their own. This misconception is in fact quite often the opposite of the reality - it takes strength of character to ask for help and a mature and realistic awareness of ones own personal limitations. Those who are strong enough to ask for help clearly demonstrate a strength of character and commitment to successfully achieving their goals that is missing in those who are too worried about what others may think of them.

A second common reason for not wanting to ask for support is this:

Addicts tend to think that they don't really need support and that they can manage well on their own.

If you are one of these addicts then consider this - If you know best and don't need that level of support, how come you are still smoking? There is obviously something missing from your game plan. Your attempts to stop smoking without support have not worked, otherwise you would not be still trying to find a way to stop. Consider this next question carefully if you are a nicotine addict, and feel that you don't really need support:

What if it is only this missing support that has prevented you from succeeding in the past?

Surely using all available support has got to be worth a try!

A third reason why addicts may be reluctant to seek support:

Addicts have a greater than average tendency to be 'people pleasers', and don't want to ask for assistance in case the person they ask regards them as a bit of a nuisance.

They also might be afraid that the person they ask to help them may say no, and then they would have to deal with the discomfort of feeling rejected. They worry about all of this and then come to the conclusion that they don't really need help and that they will manage well on their own. Let me make it clear now - if you are one of these people you are simply deluding yourself in order to avoid discomfort. Yes, it's that little 'voice' again trying to keep you from feeling discomfort, and to hell with the price you have to pay!

The key message here is that if you are reluctant to seek support that's OK, it is a normal enough reaction, but don't let your discomfort stop you from asking, because to do so is to severely reduce your chances of Succeeding.

Everyone who is addicted to nicotine needs support to help them Overcome their addiction and to think that you are an exception to this rule is to fall foul of your own denial. If you find yourself thinking that you will be regarded as weak for asking for help, remember, it is the weak who are afraid to ask for help. They are afraid of what others may think. It is the strong who ask for help, showing strength of character that allows them to ask in spite of what others may think.

If you find yourself thinking that you know best and that you can manage just as well on your own, ask yourself this question: "If I am so smart and so self supporting, how come I'm still a smoker?"

If you find yourself thinking that you don't want to be a nuisance, promise yourself that you will feel the discomfort and ask for support anyway. You know that if the person you are asking is any kind of friend at all they will be only too glad to help you, After all, if they were to ask you, wouldn't you be supportive of them?

Of course you would. Wouldn't you be flattered that you were the person they chose to trust with something that could mean the difference between life and death? As you have probably gathered by now, using all the following support structures is of the utmost importance and there is no good reason not to, despite what your little 'voice' tries to tell you!

Just before you look at the following strategies, take note that you do not need to remember or act on them straight away. In the end section of the book, they will all be summarized in the form of a simple to follow 'battle plan'.

Know this for certain:

If you choose to use all of the support structures you can be absolutely certain that you will become an ex smoker. If you do not, then you may well smoke again. You have been warned!

In the next chapter, we will examine the strategies that will, if utilized, make failing to stop smoking even more difficult than succeeding!

CHAPTER 5 – SUCCESS STRATEGIES

1. **Tell absolutely everyone you know, that you have stopped smoking and tell them that this time you have it conquered. Tell them, also, that you know that you will never smoke again and if you ever do, you will be a fool. Better still, tell any rivals, or Enemies or work colleagues who you don't get on too well with!**

You don't need to be a psychologist to work out the reasoning behind this ploy. The more people you tell and the more determined you appear to them to become a non smoker, then the more difficult it will be for you to start smoking again. Sometimes, when the going gets rough, the thought of losing face in front of a work colleague, or your mum, or your boss, may be the thing that keeps you from smoking until that particular bad patch passes.

The same logic applies to telling a rival or enemy. The effect is even more pronounced because the loss of face appears even more severe. You may, of course, feel frightened to take this course of action in case you do fail, but if this thought of losing face does frighten you, then what better incentive to stay stopped? Go on, make that commitment!

2. **Ask all of your friends, colleagues and relations to support you by firstly, taking you seriously and secondly, by never offering you a cigarette.**

Again, the value of this tactic is self evident, If your associates don't take you seriously then it makes it easier for you to relapse in their presence. A word of warning here. Some of you will find that no matter how much you implore some people to support you, they will not take you seriously. Some individuals may actually even encourage you to smoke again.

These individuals sound uncannily like your little 'voice', and their problem may be that they feel threatened by your resolve to beat your nicotine addiction. They may be people who have little or no belief in their own ability to stop smoking and don't want you to succeed for fear that they will be left behind. They are clearly, very self interested and should be regarded with the same disdain that you have for your little 'voice'.

Sometimes these individuals are non smokers or ex smokers and their problem may well be that they cannot bear to see someone making good or succeeding at something. Quite often this is because many such individuals feel bad about themselves and try to compensate for their negative feelings by trying to drag others down to their level.

An alternative theory as to why these people would act with such blatant disregard for the welfare of others is that they may be ignorant of the seriousness of the situation. Although lets face it, if you don't know by now that smoking is a ridiculously dangerous and stupid thing to do, then you will probably never know!

Ask yourself this question if you find someone trying to encourage you to smoke, and you are wondering if it is because they just don't know any better:

Would they encourage their own children to smoke?   - I don't think so!

If you do come across one of these individuals who try to talk you or joke you into smoking, or if they continue to offer you cigarettes after you have asked them not to, assert yourself by taking them to one side and telling them straight that you are deadly serious about stopping, that you expect them to be a bit more supportive, and if they feel that they still can't take you seriously then ask them frankly to stay out of your way. If after all that they still don't respond, I think it is safe to say that you have either got yourself an enemy, or possibly a friend who is just exceptionally stupid!

3. **Ask someone you respect and see often, to be your stop smoking sponsor.**

Ask them to check on you twice a day (noon and 8,00pm are good times) to see how you are getting on. Ask them to read this book or teach them the basic principles in order that they know best how to offer you support. The knowledge that your sponsor is going to contact you on a regular basis for the first couple of weeks will help you to maintain a high level of motivation, and this will be particularly useful if you encounter any rough times. It is important to stress to your sponsor just how serious you are, in order that they can commit themselves to maintaining regular contact with you.

If you find that the person you have chosen is turning out to be unreliable then quickly choose someone else in addition to them, because for the first two or three weeks in particular, this high level of support could mean the difference between success and failure.

Once again I would like to remind you of the importance of following this guidance. To ignore it because you think you know best or because it is too much hassle is to plan for failure.

4. On an A4 sheet of paper, draw two lines of seven squares. Divide each square into four quarters, each quarter to represent a quarter day, for a period of two weeks. Use a marker to color in each successful quarter day that you have not smoked, until you reach the end of the two weeks.

Then make a similar chart for the next two weeks, except mark it in days. At the successful completion of these four weeks (hurray! your first month) make a chart for one month and mark it in full days. By the completion of this second month you will find that you no longer need to keep counting the days, as the vast majority of your symptoms will be at a low level, and many of them will have gone completely.

If, however, you find that you are a low pain threshold individual and you would like to make another daily chart for the following month, then please feel free to do so. The bottom line is that the more support you get, from any source, the more likely you are to succeed.

5. Reward yourself. In your first week reward yourself with a little treat for every successful day completed.

This could be something like buying your favorite magazine to read in bed at the end of a successful smoke free day, or a special food, or a favorite drink at your supper time. It could be, for example, putting the money that you have saved from not buying cigarettes into a jar, in order to save for a bigger treat, or perhaps a nice bunch of flowers for yourself.

Anything, in fact, that will remind you that you are a success and as such deserve these little treats. Treating yourself like this is a good way to reinforce your initial commitment to stopping smoking by allowing you to feel like the winner that you have now become.

6. Each night as you go to bed tell yourself out loud:

"Today I have won the battle with my little 'voice'. I am strong and successful. Tomorrow I will win the battle also, no matter what comes my way."

On getting out of bed each morning tell yourself *"Yesterday I was a success, today I will be a success also, no matter what comes my way."*

This simple motivational technique will help to ensure that you recognize just how well you are doing and will encourage you to stay on track on any given day.

Don't worry about how you are going to remember all this information. In the final chapter this entire book will be summarized into a simple, easy to follow 'battle plan' which you can follow in your daily life, until you are strong enough to go it alone.

7. Do not let yourself get too hungry, angry, lonely or tired.

Any of these four conditions can leave you feeling exceptionally Vulnerable, even if you have only been exposed to them for a short time. Keep his in your mind with the help of the acronym H.A.L.T. (Hungry, Angry, Lonely, Tired.)

Let's take a brief look at each of these conditions separately:

HUNGRY - as mentioned before, the feelings of hunger are remarkably similar to the feelings of nicotine withdrawal. That being the case, it makes good sense not to add to these withdrawal feelings by letting yourself get hungry.

ANGRY - When people get angry there is a tendency for two things to happen. Firstly, rational judgement can disappear and the decision to not smoke can suddenly no longer seem to be overly important. Secondly, angry people are stressed people and there is barely a smoker alive who doesn't automatically reach for a cigarette when feeling stressed. This combination of high stress and impaired judgement is an obvious a recipe for disaster, Simply being aware of this potential failing point will go some way towards allowing you to successfully overcome your anger, without having to resort to smoking.

LONELY - Loneliness is one of the most powerful of our emotions. If you allow yourself to become lonely or isolated you will run the risk of suffering from self pity, or 'the poor me's' as it is widely know in the addiction field. Self pity, just like anger, can lead to a distorted perspective of what is important, and subsequently you could find yourself saying something like, "Sure nobody really cares, what's the point of stopping smoking, aren't we all going to die sooner or later anyway?" Again, this is just you little 'voice' taking advantage of your temporary vulnerability. In order to avoid this situation, try to stay around people as much as possible, particularly in the first two or three weeks.

TIRED - Again, just like hunger, the symptoms of tiredness are remarkably similar to nicotine withdrawal. Try to rest as often as possible, get plenty of sleep and take as many early nights as you can, particularly in the first two or three weeks when you will be at your most vulnerable.

8. Be aware that sometime in the future it is likely that you will have to face a major crisis.

You may contract a serious illness or be involved in a car accident; you may suffer the breakdown of a long term relationship or lose your job. Life can be very cruel sometimes, but no matter what happens to you, you do not need to smoke.

Smoking will not make things better and if you tell yourself that it will be OK to smoke if a major crisis comes along, then you are doomed to fail. Life being what it is, you can be sure that sooner or later you *will* have a crisis of one sort or another to face.

You need to decide *now* that if, or when your crisis occurs, you are not going to smoke.

The value of implementing these support structures cannot be over emphasized. Setting up and using these structures will certainly result in you successfully stopping smoking. To ignore them or to choose only the ones you feel most comfortable with will significantly reduce your chances of becoming a non smoker.

Before we move on to look at your stop smoking 'battle plan', we need to address the problem of weight gain that is often associated with stopping smoking. If the thought of putting on weight is a significant concern for you, then let me assure you that if any weight gain problems do occur, they can be sorted out quickly and effectively by using the information in the following chapter.

CHAPTER 6 - WEIGHT MANAGEMENT

One of the most frequently used excuses for starting smoking again goes something like this: "Oh, I was doing ever so well, but my weight just soared and I had to start smoking again before I looked like a beached whale."

Rubbish! As you now know, there is never any valid reason to resume smoking. Weight gain may occasionally be an issue, but it is certainly a resolvable issue.

Just because you stop smoking, it doesn't necessarily follow that you will put on weight. There are two factors to be considered here. First of all your metabolism. It has been reported that a for a *minority* of individuals, stopping smoking can lead to a *small* change in their metabolic rate. What this means in layman's terms is that a little more of the food you eat is converted into fat and stored on your body.

This is obviously not good news for you if you are concerned about weight gain, but it is not as bad as it might at first appear. For a start, this phenomenon only occurs in a minority of individuals, and furthermore the changed metabolic rate is normally quite small. Here is the main reason that some people put on weight when they stop smoking:

NICOTINE WITHDRAWAL PRODUCES FEELINGS SIMILAR TO HUNGER!

Hunger is another of those feelings that is under the control of your little 'voice' and it knows, of course, that the solution to the pain of hunger is to eat.

Lets look at another conscious / unconscious dialogue:

U: (having felt the pain of withdrawal) "Have a smoke"

C: "No I have stopped smoking."

U: "Look, I am absolutely gasping, have a smoke for goodness sake!"

C: "No chance, I am staying stopped"

U: (realising that for the time being it is not going to win, starts to look for alternative pain relieving strategies.) "Mmmm... this feels very like being hungry, perhaps food will take away the discomfort - I'll have something to eat."

C: (Not having made any resolutions at all with regards to eating, agrees immediately) "OK."

Off you go to the fridge, only to find that after stuffing yourself you still have the feeling of withdrawal, which as you know, feels very similar to hunger. Your unconscious is still not happy of course and so the whole process starts over again:

Pain >> Eat >> Still pain >> Eat again >> Still pain >> Eat again

And that's the way it goes, on and on, until you find yourself the size of a baby elephant.

The good news is that it doesn't have to be that way. There is a simple three part formula that determines whether or not you put on weight and it is this:

1. If you consume more calories than you burn off, then you will put on weight.

2. If you consume the same amount of calories that you burn off then your weight will remain constant.

3. If you consume less calories than you burn off you will lose weight.

Now with this knowledge to hand it becomes easy to formulate a plan that will allow you to indulge (if you want to) in filling your stomach when you feel the pain of withdrawal, without having to suffer the end result of putting on more weight.

This strategy can take one of two basic forms:

1. **Eat more food but without consuming additional calories, or:**

2. **Increase the amount of calories that you burn off each day.**

Let's look at strategy 1 first.

You are going to want to eat a lot more, particularly in the early days, so in order to do this without putting on any weight you have to increase the amount of food you eat in terms of volume, yet still maintain roughly the same calorific intake. This is not as difficult to achieve as it sounds. If you agree to modify your diet from the moment you stop smoking, not only will you find it possible to maintain your normal weight, but you are almost certainly going to be benefiting nutritionally.

This is because; (unless you are already particularly fussy about eating healthily) you are going to improve your diet enormously by introducing plenty of fresh fruit and vegetables and by cutting down significantly on your fat intake.

Below you will find a list of common foods and their fat and calorific values. All you have to do is to swap foods that you now eat regularly with a high calorific / fat content for those with a low (or at least lower) value.

Before looking at the food lists, bear in mind these few simple rules. Adherence to them will make a significant difference to your overall fat, and subsequently calorie, consumption.

> Don't eat any fried foods. (Deep or shallow fried.) Boil, poach, bake or grill instead.

> Don't eat out for a few weeks. (A typical Indian or Chinese take away for example, can easily contain over 2,000 calories!)

> Avoid sweets and sugar based treats. (cakes, buns, soft drinks etc.

> Check the nutritional labels on all packaged foods and avoid any that are high in fat (i.e. 10 per cent or more)

> Use your favorite fruits and vegetables as comfort foods, as most fruit and vegetables are OK in terms of fat and calories. (Check them against the following lists).

> Drink plenty of water. This is important for two reasons - first, it helps to detoxify you by flushing the poisons from your system. This will include the removal of nicotine from your body. Second, drinking plenty of wate

will take away some of your feelings of hunger and therefore make it easier for you to eat less, and still feel full up.

> Study this list of common foods and choose an assortment that you like. Substitute some of your usual higher fat foods for the foods that you have selected from the list below. Check that you are making a significant calorie difference by ensuring that your new choices of food have a lower calorific value than the ones you have swapped them for.

Remember, this food watching business is only necessary if you are one of those people who find themselves constantly at the fridge door when stopping smoking! The following lists are a rough guide to the amount of calories and fat that you can expect to find in certain foods:

FRUIT		FAT (g)	CALORIES
APPLES	(1)	0	70
AVOCADO	(1)	36	370
BANANA	(1)	TRACE	85
CANTALOUPE	(1)	TRACE	80
CHERRIES	(1 CUP)	TRACE	65
DATES	(1 CUP)	TRACE	505
GRAPEFRUIT	(1)	TRACE	50
GRAPES	(1 CUP)	TRACE	100
ORANGES	(1)	TRACE	60
PEACHES	(1)	TRACE	35
PEARS	(1)	TRACE	30
PLUMS	(1)	TRACE	25
STRAWBERRIES	(1 CUP)	1	55

BREADS AND CEREALS	FAT (g)	CALORIES
WHITE BREAD (1 SLICE)	1	70
WHOLE-WHEAT (1 SLICE)	1	65
CORNFLAKES (1 CUP)	TRACE	110
FLOUR WHITE (1 CUP)	1	400
CHEESE (1 CUP)	25	475
MUFFINS (1)	5	135
NOODLES (1 CUP)	2	200
PIZZA (1 SLICE)	6	180
RICE, BROWN (1 CUP)	3	748
SPAGHETTI (1 CUP)	10	285
SHREDDED WHEAT (1)	1	100
WAFFLES (1)	9	240

....

MEAT	FAT (g)	CALORIES
BACON (1 SLICE, GRILLED)	4	47
BEEF (ROAST 3 0Z)	36	390
BEEF (CORNED 3 OZ)	10	185
BEEF (STEAK 3 OZ, GRILLED)	27	330
CHICKEN (3 OZ, ROASTED)	17	250
CHILLI CON CARNE (1 CUP)	15	325
LAMB CHOP (GRILLED, 4 OZ)	35	480
LIVER (LAMBS, 3 OZ)	12	260
PORK CHOP (1)	21	280
PORK SAUSAGE (3 OZ)	44	475
TURKEY (ROASTED, 3 OZ)	15	265
VEAL CUTLET (GRILLED, 3 OZ)	9	185

EGGS AND DAIRY PRODUCE	Fat(gr)	(kCal)
EGGS - BOILED (1)	6	75
SCRAMBLED (1)	8	110
MILK (FULL FAT, 1 CUP)	9	160
MILK (SEMI SKIMMED 1 CUP)	5	145
CHEESE (CHEDDAR, 1 OZ)	9	115
(COTTAGE, 1 CUP)	1	170
CREAM (WHIPPING, 1 TB SPOON)	6	45
CREAM (LIGHT, 1 TB SPOON)	3	30
CUSTARD (BAKED, 1 CUP)	14	285
ICE CREAM 1 CUP	18	300

....

FISH PRODUCTS	Fat(gr)	kCal
COD (GRILLED 3 OZ)	5	170
FISHCAKES (FRIED, 2)	8	175
FISH FINGERS (FRIED, 5)	10	200
HADDOCK (FRIED, 3 OZ)	5	135
LOBSTER (STEAMED, 1)	2	184
OYSTERS (6)	2	80
PRAWNS 3 OZ	1	110
SARDINES TINNED 3 OZ	9	180
TUNA TINNED 3 OZ	7	170

VEGETABLES		FAT	kCal
BEANS, BROAD	1 CUP	TRACE	140
KIDNEY	1 CUP	1	230
BEETROOT	1 CUP	TRACE	68
BROCCOLI	1 CUP	TRACE	45
BRUSSELS SPROUTS	1 CUP	TRACE	60
CABBAGE	1 CUP	TRACE	40
CARROTS	(RAW)	TRACE	45
CAULIFLOWER	1 CUP	TRACE	30
CELERY	1 STICK	TRACE	5
LENTILS	1 CUP	TRACE	212
LETTUCE	1	TRACE	56
MUSHROOMS (TINNED)		TRACE	12
ONIONS, COOKED, 1 CUP)		TRACE	80
PARSNIPS (STEAMED, 1 CUP)		1	95
PEAS (CANNED, 1 CUP)		TRACE	68
PEPPERS (RAW, 1)		TRACE	25
POTATOES (BAKED)		TRACE	100
POTATOES (CHIPS, 10)		7	155
POTATOES (CREAMED)		12	230
POTATO CRISPS 10		7	110
SPINACH (STEAMED)		TRACE	26
SWEETCORN (STEAMED)		1	92
TOMATOES, (RAW,)		TRACE	30
TURNIPS, (STEAMED)		TRACE	40

If you have had a good look at the above list you will have discovered how easy it can be to substitute high calorie foods for those foods with a much lower calorie content, If you choose to make this substitution on a daily basis you can easily keep yourself from feeling hunger by increasing the volume of the food you eat whilst maintaining or even reducing your calorie intake.

A second strategy for keeping your weight in check is to simply increase the amount of calories you burn each day. This can be achieved by increasing the amount of exercise you do on a daily basis. Remember, excess calories will be stored on your body as fat, so ideally you will combine both techniques of diet modification and exercise for a doubly effective approach.

Now let's take a look at strategy 2:

The following table tells you how many calories you can expect to burn by completing certain exercises.

This table relates to an individual who weighs seventy kg. If you are lighter than this you will burn off slightly less calories during each exercise and if you are heavier you will burn off slightly more - about ten percent more or less for each difference of 7 kg.

Please consult your doctor before starting any new form of exercise or before significantly increasing current levels of activity.

CALORIES PER HOUR **(APPROXIMATIONS)**	
BADMINTON	500
BASKETBALL	630
BOXING	800
BRICKLAYING	260
CALLISTHENICS	350 - 600
CIRCUIT TRAINING	600
CYCLING:	
SLOW	275
MEDIUM	410
FAST	600
DANCING:	
SLOW	400
FAST	600

FENCING	650
FISHING	300
GARDENING	450
GOLFING	350
GYMNASTICS	300
HORSE RIDING	330
HOUSEWORK	300
ICE HOCKEY	600
MOUNTAIN CLIMBING	600
MOWING	400
TABLE TENNIS	475
SKIPPING (HARD)	800
RUNNING:	
SLOW	700
MEDIUM	950
FAST	1150
SAWING HARDWOOD	600
SEX	375 - 600
SKIING	600
SKATING	500 - 1000
SCUBA DIVING	1000
SOCCER	775
SQUASH	650
SWIMMING	350 - 900
TENNIS	500
WALKING	200 - 500
WALKING UPSTAIRS	600 - 1100
WEIGHT TRAINING	500
WRESTLING	900

These figures in the food and exercise tables give you a rough guide as to what you will be able to eat in addition to or as a substitute for, your normal diet. For example, if you were to have an hour brisk walk in addition to your normal daily routine then you could safely eat extra food to the value of 300

400 calories without putting on any additional weight. Perhaps a portion of chips or a few ounces of roast beef.

Alternatively, If you were to substitute one portion of about 30 chips, (465 calories) you could exchange it for say, a cup of creamed potatoes, 2 sticks of celery, 6 oysters and 1 banana and still be eating 60 calories less! There really is no need to go hungry, just modify your diet and increase your daily exercise and you should have little or no problem in maintaining your current weight.

If you choose to put enough thought and effort into this whole process, you could quite easily even lose weight, in addition to stopping smoking!

As with all the techniques you have encountered so far in this book, the real secret of successful weight management is to make a decision and stick to it. Decide on what way you want your weight to go, work out how to achieve it, monitor your progress by regular weighing, and keep on adjusting your dietary and exercise plan until you achieve the result that you want. It really can, and will, be that easy.

If you have taken on board all the principles and knowledge contained in this book, you are now ready to begin the process of stopping smoking.

The next and final chapter will contain all the information that you need to be successful, condensed into a simple to use 'battle plan'.

CHAPTER 7 - THE 'BATTLE PLAN'

Right then - this is it, the last chapter before you becomes a nonsmoker!

What this section is going to do is to sort out all the practical information from the rest of the book and put it into the form of a simple plan of instructions from which you can work on a daily basis.

When you finish this section you can take your last smoke (if you want one that is!) and then begin your journey into the land of the non smoker. You now have everything that you need to be a success and absolutely no valid excuses to fail. I won't wish you luck - you wont need it.

What you will need however, is to make a resolution to keep plodding away with all the techniques discussed in this book until you find yourself in a position where you feel confident enough to continue on your own, without the need for assistance from your support structures.

This whole stopping smoking process will start off feeling a little difficult at first but with each passing day your journey will become easier.

It is of the utmost importance that you hang in there during any rough patches that you may encounter because you can be absolutely certain that they will pass. You will help them to pass easier and quicker by employing the tactics you have learned from this book.

If you do so, you will find that in what seems like no time at all you will regard yourself not just as someone who is trying to stop smoking, but as an ex smoker.

If I was to try and identify the single most important piece of advice that will best help you to succeed, I would say it would be this:

NO MATTER WHAT HAPPENS, DON'T PICK UP A CIGARETTE.

Remember, once again that there is simply no valid excuse, not even something as painful as the death of a loved one, and considering smoking for anything less is simply to admit defeat to that little 'voice' in your head.

THE 'BATTLE PLAN'

1. **IN WRITING,** state that you understand and admit that you are a nicotine addict. If you haven't already done this *DO IT RIGHT NOW!*

2. **IN WRITING**, state that you are going to stop smoking at the end of this book and that you will never smoke again. Sign this declaration and put it on a wall that you will see every day. Your bathroom is a good place to put it. If you haven't already done this, *DO IT RIGHT NOW!*

3. **SAY OUT LOUD** to yourself that you will follow all of the instructions and use all of the tactics in this book, whenever requested or necessary. *DO THIS NOW!*

4. **REMEMBER** that you will always be addicted to nicotine, therefore there will be no time when it is OK to have a smoke.

5. **AGREE** to pay the price of sometimes tolerating some discomfort and know that not only will this discomfort soon pass, but also that it is a very small price to pay to become a nonsmoker.

6. **BE AWARE** of the little 'voice'. Make it your sworn enemy and know that it doesn't care about your welfare and will constantly feed you with contrived excuses in order to make you smoke. THERE IS NO VALID EXCUSE FOR STARTING SMOKING AGAIN. If you smoke again it is always because you were conned by this 'voice' and refused to pay the price of short term discomfort.

7. **MAKE A PAIN CHART** and put it on your wall. When you feel that the going is getting a bit tough, do a head to toe body check and measure the real strength of your pain. Remember that it is seldom as bad as the little 'voice' would have you believe! *DO THIS RIGHT NOW.*

8. **REMEMBER that 'THIS TOO, SHALL PASS'**, if you hit a rough patch

9. **ONE DAY AT A TIME** when used as a pain management strategy will help to get even those of you with an extremely low pain threshold, through the roughest of patches. If necessary, you can reduce this to one hour, or even 5 minutes at a time.

10. **H.A.L.T.** Remember never to get too hungry, angry lonely or tired Do whatever it takes to avoid these emotionally vulnerable mental states.

11. **TELL EVERYONE YOU KNOW** that you are now a non smoker and that you will never smoke again. Make a particular point of telling those people who you don't get on with, or those who would like to see you fail

This tactic can sometimes mean the difference between success and failure! So go ahead - pick up the phone. *DO THIS RIGHT NOW!*

12. **ASK YOUR FRIENDS,** family and colleagues to give you all the support that they can, and to take you seriously. Tell them never to offer you a cigarette and to be patient and tolerant if you happen to experience any mood swings. ***START THIS PROCESS RIGHT NOW!***

13. **ENLIST THE SUPPORT** of someone you really respect and trust. Regard them as your stop smoking sponsor and ask them to phone you twice a day for the first few weeks to check on your progress. Give them a copy of this book to read, or talk them through the main points, in order that they are in a position to better support you. IF YOU FIND YOU ARE TEMPTED TO SMOKE, pick up the phone and talk to your sponsor and if they are not available then don't use that as an excuse to smoke, just talk to someone else, or wait until your sponsor does becomes available. **ASK SOMEONE TO BE YOUR SPONSOR RIGHT NOW!**

14. **CHART YOUR SUCCESS.** Make a daily, weekly and monthly success chart as described in the chapter on support. Fill this chart in every day and know that with each passing successful day your symptoms are reducing and your chances of succeeding are becoming greater and greater. It is only a matter of time now before you can call yourself an ex smoker! ***DO THIS RIGHT NOW!***

15. **REWARD YOURSELF** every day for the first two weeks, and every week for the first two or three months. Something small for the daily rewards and something a little more significant for the end of each successful week.

16. **MONITOR YOUR WEIGHT** and adjust by means of diet and / or exercise, as necessary.

17.   **MOTIVATE YOURSELF** by verbalizing your daily success and daily intentions. Do this every night and every morning, as described in the support strategies chapter.

18.   **CELEBRATE BIG TIME** your new life as an ex smoker at the end of about the third or fourth month. This will probably be around the time when you will start to feel comfortable with the idea that you are now an ex smoker and not just someone who is trying to give up.

19.   **REMEMBER** that for the next year or two (or perhaps even for ever) you are still going to hear that little 'voice'. Only on the odd occasion and only quite weakly, but you must be aware of its constant presence because if you are at any stage to light up a cigarette, then you will revive this little monster to its former strength and you may well have to start from scratch. After a few months there is not really going to be any serious problem staying stopped, provided that:

NO MATTER WHAT HAPPENS, UNDER ANY CIRCUMSTANCES, YOU DO NOT TAKE A CIGARETTE.

CHAPTER 8 - WELCOME TO YOUR NEW LIFE

OK, that's it then. If you have finished setting up all the above support systems then your time has arrived.

Finally, throw away any remaining cigarettes that you may have, follow all the above instructions.

Thank you for reading *Easiest Way To Stop Smoking*.

David Walters

Printed in Great Britain
by Amazon

27086753R00047